Patient Management Problems in Psychiatry

for the MRCPsych II exam

D1634686

Albert Michael (editor)

Consultant Psychiatrist
West Suffolk Hospital
Bury St. Edmunds
UK

This publication is presented as a service to
psychiatry by Eli Lilly and Company Ltd.

SCIENCE PRESS

Published by Science Press Limited, 34–42 Cleveland Street, London W1P 6LB, UK

http://current-science-group.com/

© Science Press Ltd 2000

British Library Cataloguing-in Publication Data.

A catalogue record for this book is available from the British Library.

ISBN 1-85873-905-5

This publication is presented as a service to psychiatry by Eli Lilly and Company Ltd. Sponsorship of this copy does not imply the sponsor's agreement or otherwise with the views expressed herein.

Although every effort has been made to ensure that drug doses and other information are presented accurately in this publication, the ultimate responsibility rests with the prescribing physician. Neither the publishers nor the authors can be held responsible for errors or for any consequences arising from the use of information contained herein. Any product mentioned in this publication should be used in accordance with the prescribing information prepared by the manufacturers. No claims or endorsements are made for any drug or compound at present under clinical investigation.

Project editor: Mark Knowles
Typesetter: Simon Banister
Designer: Claire Huntley
Production: David Forrest
Printed in the UK by Newnorth Print Ltd.

Contents

Contributors

Alex Baldacchino MD, MPhil, DAB, MRCPsych.
Senior Lecturer/Honorary Consultant Psychiatrist, St George's Medical School.

Michael Blows MBChB, MRCP, MRCPsych.
Consultant in Child and Adolescent Psychiatry, Bury St Edmunds.

Donald Bermingham MBBCh, BAO, MRCPsych.
Consultant Psychiatrist, Hinchingbrooke Healthcare NHS Trust, Huntingdon.

Jon Darley MA, MBChB, MRCPsych.
Consultant in Old Age Psychiatry, West Suffolk Hospital, Bury St Edmunds.

Chess Denman MBBS, MRCPsych.
Consultant Psychiatrist in Psychological Treatments, Cambridge.

Harsha Fernando MBBS, MRCPsych.
Consultant Psychiatrist and Postgraduate Tutor, Peterborough.

Justine Gardner MRCPsych.
Consultant in Rehabilitation Psychiatry, Hellesdon Hospital, Norwich.

Jonathan Hillam MRCPsych.
Consultant in Old Age Psychiatry, King's Lynn & Wisbech Hospitals NHS Trust.

Luk W Ho BA, MBBCh, MRCPsych.
Specialist Registrar in Psychiatry, Cambridge.

Anthony Holland MBBS, MRCP, MRCPsych.
University Lecturer/Honorary Consultant Psychiatrist, Cambridge.

Neil Hunt MA, MD, MRCPsych.
Consultant Psychiatrist, Cambridge.

Mervyn London MBChB, MRCPsych.
Consultant Psychiatrist, Cambridge.

Albert Michael MBBS, MD, DPM, MRCPsych.
Consultant Psychiatrist, West Suffolk Hospital, Bury St Edmunds.

Richard O'Flynn MRCPsych.
Consultant in General Adult Psychiatry, West Suffolk Hospital.

Siri Robling MB BChir, MA(Cantab), MRCPsych.
Consultant in General Adult Psychiatry, West Suffolk Hospital.

Bohdan Solomka BMedSci, BMBS, MRCPsych.
Consultant in Forensic Psychiatry, The Norvic Clinic, Norwich.

Andrew F Tarbuck BMBCh, MA, MRCPsych.
Consultant in Old Age Psychiatry and Clinical Tutor in Psychiatry, Norwich.

Petrus de Vries MBChB, MRCPsych.
Clinical Research Associate and Honorary Specialist Registrar, Cambridge.

Tim Webb MBChB, MRCPsych.
Consultant in General Adult Psychiatry, West Suffolk Hospital, Bury St Edmunds.

Jo Wong MBBS, MA, MRCPsych.
Assistant Professor of Psychiatry, University of Hong Kong.

Foreword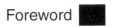

Problems of patient management, in a practical context, comprise the essence of the daily professional life of the practising psychiatrist. From a more focused perspective, patient management problems are also an important component of the MRCPsych examination, the qualifying hurdle that must be surmounted by every aspirant UK psychiatrist.

Dr Albert Michael, the editor of this volume, is a very experienced, enthusiastic and successful teacher, and is the Course Organiser for the Regional MRCPsych Part I and Part II Courses for East Anglia. He has assembled contributors who are all active teachers of psychiatric postgraduates.

The editor and the contributors to this book have devised and refined a wide-ranging and comprehensive set of problems, covering issues of management, which extend from the relatively common to areas often relatively unfamiliar to the general adult psychiatrist. They will be of value not only to MRCPsych candidates, but also to practising consultants of all specialities and all levels of experience who wish to keep abreast of current practice across the range of psychiatry, including those fields with which they have little contact. I commend this very useful volume to its readers.

Eugene S Paykel MD, FRCP, FRCPsych, FmedSci.
Professor of Psychiatry,
University of Cambridge.

Introduction ▪

The clinical examination for the Part II MRCPsych examination has two parts: the 'Individual Patient Assessment' (formerly the 'Clinical Examination') and the 'Patient Management Problems' [PMP] (formerly the 'Oral Examination'). The candidate is required to pass the clinical examination as a whole, and not necessarily each part.

In the 30-minute PMP session, two examiners present two problems each, and if time permits, a fifth one. Usually the problems are presented verbally, though some examiners have the problems written on cards. Some examiners present all the relevant information in the beginning. Others give broad problems and fill in the gaps as the candidate progresses through the management.

The candidate is expected to display a grasp of the problems presented, to recognise the difficulties and dangers that might arise, to suggest methods of investigation and management which are realistic, and to be able to present evidence from the literature for the measures they have chosen to adopt. Thus, the object is to test the candidate's judgement and skill, as well as knowledge.

The examiners usually present real problems that they themselves have encountered and found interesting or difficult to manage. Hence, the problems should be answered as if they were real situations. Candidates should listen carefully, cross-check the details with the examiner if necessary, think clearly and work through the problem methodically and systematically. It is important to avoid jumping to conclusions and candidates should not give the impression that they consider a problem too simple. The aim is to prove that, as a practitioner, the examinee will be safe and reliable, even while under pressure. As each problem is drawn from real life there should be, naturally, a way of at least assessing the situation. If the candidate feels completely lost with a question, it may be safer for them to ask to move on to the next question instead of prevaricating and wasting time.

There is no substitute for theoretical knowledge and clinical experience. Even with the best experience, candidates often find the PMP intimidating. This book aims to help them prepare for the unexpected and look systematically at a variety of problems.

Ideally, readers should try to answer each question before looking at the next, and answer all the questions in each problem before looking at the answers given in the book. Space is provided below the questions for making notes.

Examiners, problems and candidates vary; hence, I have tried to incorporate the collective wisdom of a variety of clinician trainers to provide the trainees with as varied an experience as possible. All the contributors are or have been trainees or trainers, or both, at the East Anglian Regional MRCPsych Course, Fulbourn Hospital, Cambridge.

I acknowledge with gratitude the contribution of all my colleagues without whose commitment and enthusiasm this venture would not have materialized.

You have admitted a 25-year-old man, who is managed on a depot neuroleptic for schizophrenia, for reassessment because of increasing self-neglect and social withdrawal. On admission, he tells you he has been injecting heroin daily for the past three months.

1. *How do you proceed further in the assessment?*

2. *How do you manage this patient during the admission?*

3. *How do you plan aftercare, following discharge?*

Further assessment. Assessment should include enquiries about use of alcohol and other illicit substances, psychosocial factors that may underlie the drug use, and the nature and frequency of the heroin use and risk factors arising from it, eg, from shared needles. What is the patient's motivation to change his drug use? I will consider blood tests for hepatitis and HIV.

I will ascertain whether the psychosis relapsed before or after onset of heroin use, his level of compliance with treatment and whether there are any problematic side effects from medication.

I will seek confirmation of heroin use by examining for injection sites and testing urine samples for illicit drugs, ascertain dependence on opiates by examining for signs of withdrawal, and arrange for nursing staff to monitor for withdrawal symptoms during the first 24–48 hours of admission.

Patient management during admission. One must address both the psychosis and the heroin use. Antipsychotic medication must be reviewed if there have been significant side effects or a psychotic relapse. These may be contributory factors to the heroin use.

Since the duration of his heroin use is relatively short, the preferred goal is abstinence. If the patient is dependent there are two options for detoxification – methadone mixture or symptomatic treatment. If methadone treatment is chosen, give incremental doses of methadone over the first 24–48 hours, to control objective withdrawal symptoms until a stable level is achieved. Then reduce the dose in a stepwise daily fashion until detoxified. The patient's level of dependence may not require opiates, however, there are drawbacks in introducing this patient to methadone.

Lofexidine, an alpha$_2$-adrenergic agonist, or combinations of a sedative, antidiarrhoeal and antiemetic drug can be used. I will consider immunizing the patient against hepatitis.

Aftercare, following discharge. Involve the community drug team in follow-up for psychoeducation intervention and/or ongoing treatment.

A community methadone prescription may become appropriate later if there is persistent intravenous heroin use. Naltrexone is an option, in order to reinforce abstinence.

Consider activities to replace previous drug-centred behaviours.

Community mental health team, daycare services and carers should be aware of the heroin problem and it should be a factor in the care plan.

A GP telephones you for your advice about a 28-year-old woman who gave birth to her first child three weeks ago. Her husband came to the GP, complaining that she is acting bizarrely. She is up all night, talking incessantly and her behaviour is chaotic. The health visitor is also concerned, particularly as the husband, a long-distance lorry driver, is going back to work in a few days.

1. What information would you like to have from the GP during this telephone conversation?

2. The GP asks for you to make a domiciliary visit and explains that the patient's husband will be at home and will let you in. On arrival you discover an exhausted-looking lady who can barely sit still long enough to be examined. How do you proceed?

3. You decide that the lady is probably suffering from a psychotic illness with a predominately manic presentation. She has no past psychiatric history. She appears exhausted, is unable to give a coherent account of events and is displaying a flight of ideas that suggest some very odd beliefs about the baby. How do you proceed?

Information from the GP.

- Has the GP seen the patient?
- Does the patient know her husband was consulting the GP?
- Does the woman have a known psychiatric history and if so what is it?
- Is there a family psychiatric history, of puerperal or non-puerperal illness?
- How is her physical health?
- What does the GP think is wrong?
- Is there any relevant information about the background circumstances?
- Is an appointment necessary and how urgent is this?
- Is any medication being prescribed?

Domiciliary visit. I will try to get a history from the patient, as well as from her husband, and do a mental state examination.

I will consider the differential diagnosis:

- Postnatal blues (onset of this condition is too late and the symptoms are too severe to be 'blues').
- Postnatal depression (look for depressive symptoms, especially guilt feelings).
- Postnatal psychosis: affective or schizophrenic (mixed or rapidly changing features, bizarre delusions about the baby which may or may not be mood congruent, labile affect).
- Other functional illness occurring coincidentally in the puerperium, eg, recurrent depressive episode, organic confusional state.

I will specifically assess her thoughts about the baby and the degree of risk to herself and to the baby or any other individuals, either as a result of her delusions or through neglect.

If mentally ill, decide on management, ie, outpatient/inpatient.

Procedure, following diagnosis. I will discuss my views with her husband. This patient would need further assessment and treatment in hospital. Outpatient treatment will be unsafe for the patient as well as for the baby, particularly if her husband is going to be away. I will discuss with her husband about child-care arrangements. If I have the option of a mother and baby unit that can safely take the baby, I will consider this. Most acute psychiatric wards are often not safe places to have a baby, particularly when the mother is so unwell. If there is any suspicion of the patient having thoughts of harming the baby, I will ensure the baby is not brought in with her.

I will try to explain to the patient what is happening. Even though she may be very frightened, she may be able to comprehend the information better than she appears to.

In discussion with the ward team, we will decide on a management plan, including medication and level of observation. We will plan to reintroduce the baby to the mother safely, once she is recovering.

You have a 23-year-old male patient on your ward. He has been treated for the last three months for a first episode of schizophrenia. He continues to have auditory hallucinations commenting on his actions. After watching a television programme he is convinced he is the Son of God. He is not improving despite taking haloperidol 10 mg qds and having previously been treated with chlorpromazine. His self-care seems to be deteriorating. How will you manage this case?

This patient apparently has a treatment-resistant schizophrenic illness. I would review his diagnosis and treatment and find out the reasons for resistance to treatment. I will also consider psychosocial interventions.

Review of diagnosis. I would review his history, do a mental state examination and a physical examination and seek further information from the nursing team, family and his GP. I will consider the possibility of an affective disorder, particularly in view of the grandiosity. I have to exclude organic causes such as complex partial seizures and drug-induced psychosis in this young patient. I will look for atypical signs, such as clouding of consciousness. A urine drug screen and EEG should be considered. Further failure to confirm diagnosis or make progress would warrant a CT brain scan.

Review of drug treatment. This patient has been treated with an adequate dose of oral antipsychotic medication, ie, 40 mg of haloperidol daily. Up to 20% of in-patients may be non-compliant with medication [1]. Reasons for non-compliance include side effects, particularly akathisia and lack of insight. Compliance with medication may be enhanced by a change to either a syrup or depot preparation. Depots also have the advantage of avoiding first-pass metabolism. The dosage of haloperidol could be increased within BNF limits. EPS, if present, may be controlled with antimuscarinic drugs. I will also consider changing over to a new-generation antipsychotic. They have a lower incidence of EPS and they help treatment resistant positive and negative symptoms of schizophrenia [2].

Perpetuating factors. I will look out for evidence of high expressed emotion (high-EE) which can worsen schizophrenic symptoms [3] and also for secondary gain from being in hospital (eg, avoiding a difficult home situation). If high-EE is present, family therapy to reduce high-EE and education of carers could help the current episode and also help prevent future hospitalization [4].

Psychosocial interventions. Psychological approaches such as cognitive behavioural therapy for delusions and hallucinations are worth trying in this patient [5]. Occupational therapy, including sheltered work, should be made use of.

References.

1. Bebbington PE. **The content and context of compliance.** *Int Clin Psychopharmacol* 1995, **9**(Suppl 5):41–50.

2. Marder S. **An approach to treatment resistant schizophrenia.** *Br J Psychiatry* 1999, **174**(Suppl 37):19–21.

3. Vaughn C, Leff JP. **The influence of family and social factors on the course of psychiatric illness.** *Br J Psychiatry* 1976, **129**:125–137.

4. Kavanagh DJ. **Recent developments in expressed emotion in schizophrenia.** *Br J Psychiatry* 1992, **160**:601–620.

5. Chadwick P, Birchwood M. **The omnipotence of voices. A cognitive approach to auditory hallucinations.** *Br J Psychiatry* 1994, **164**:190–201.

Mrs Smith is a 79-year-old widow who has four children, two of whom live abroad. She lives alone in a large Victorian house that has an air of 'faded grandeur'. She has a substantial portfolio of investments, and also owns property abroad. She has become increasingly forgetful over the past 12–18 months. Mrs Smith's solicitor met Mrs Smith and one of her children who, increasingly concerned about her mother's ability to manage her affairs, had arranged the meeting. The solicitor contacted Mrs Smith's GP, asking for his views on her mental capacity. The GP contacts you because he feels that, because his patient appears to be suffering from a degree of dementia, an expert opinion is required.

Financial affairs

The issue is the medico-legal concept of mental capacity. To address this, one has to assess the patient's capacity to manage her financial affairs and to make an Enduring Power of Attorney (EPA). The legal tests of capacity for the two are different, and should be considered separately. The initial step will be a full psychiatric assessment, including a detailed history, mental state examination and a detailed cognitive function assessment.

Capacity to manage financial affairs. The assessment of one's capacity to manage one's own property and affairs is not well defined. Hence, each case requires individual consideration. In addition to the initial assessment, information about the nature and complexity of Mrs Smith's affairs will be needed to assess her grasp of her own financial affairs. I will also consider if she has been managing her affairs successfully, eg, paying bills, avoiding debts, etc. In general, Mrs Smith, who has extensive property and affairs, will require a greater degree of cognitive ability than someone with less complex affairs.

Capacity to make an EPA. An EPA is a deed in which one person (the donor) gives one or more persons (the attorney[s]) authority to act in the donor's name and behalf in relation to the donor's property and financial affairs. In order to make a valid EPA, the patient must be willing to have such a document drawn up, and agree to sign it of her own volition. She should be capable of understanding that:

i) unless she stipulates otherwise, her attorney(s) will be able to assume complete authority over her affairs,

ii) unless she stipulates otherwise, her attorney(s) will be able to do anything with her property and capital that she herself could have done,

iii) the EPA will continue if she should become mentally incapable, and

iv) should she become mentally incapable, the power will be irrevocable without confirmation by the Court of Protection (Re: K, Re: F, 1988).

She can choose her attorney(s). Relatives can contest the choice of attorney(s) and the validity of the EPA. Hence, clear documentation and record keeping are important. Appointing more than one attorney may reduce the risk of exploitation. In contentious cases, independent, trustworthy person(s) such as solicitor(s) may be appointed as attorney(s). If she is incapable of managing her affairs, and yet has capacity to make a valid EPA, the EPA would be registered with the Court of Protection immediately following its execution.

If she is cognitively so impaired that she cannot make an EPA (or should she decline to make an EPA) and should she also be incapable of administering her affairs, then her relatives or her solicitor can apply to the Court of Protection for the appointment of a receiver. A Medical Certificate (Form CP3) would be required.

Further reading.

The Law Society and The BMA. *Assessment of Mental Capacity: Guidance for Doctors and Lawyers*. London: BMA; 1995.

Delirium 05

You are the duty psychiatrist and are called to a surgical ward to assess a 45-year-old male lorry driver, who had an emergency appendicectomy three days ago. He has become confused, agitated and aggressive.

1. *How would you assess this case? What are your differential diagnoses?*

2. *You have established the most likely cause is alcohol withdrawal. How do you manage this case?*

3. *What role could the Mental Health Act play if the patient refuses to remain in hospital and refuses treatment?*

Differential diagnoses. I would be looking for the differential diagnoses of an acute confusional state. I would review the case notes for any relevant past medical history, physical examination, laboratory investigation reports, full blood count, gamma-GT etc. I will review the nursing notes and the observation charts looking for evidence of infection, dehydration, retention of urine and increasing nocturnal confusion or evidence of earlier signs of alcohol or drug withdrawal.

I would look for relevant past psychiatric disorders and use of alcohol and drugs. I will look for a collateral history from the GP's referral letter; alternatively I will ask members of staff to contact the family and, in particular, to contact the GP, looking for a background history with particular emphasis on drug or alcohol use.

Management of alcohol withdrawal delirium. The initial management will include:

- Providing adequate nursing support.
- Using parenteral benzodiazepines judiciously, to achieve quick sedation and make the situation safe.
- Avoiding use of phenothiazine antipsychotics due to risk of inducing seizures.
- Maintaining adequate hydration.
- Instituting parenteral, high-potency vitamins.
- Nursing in well-lit side room.
- Possibly transfer to psychiatric ward if not manageable on an acute surgical ward.

Further management will include:

- Detoxification with reducing dose of oral benzodiazepines.
- Diagnosis and treatment of any concurrent infection.
- Examination for primary and secondary mental illness such as anxiety or depression.
- Liaison with the community alcohol team during follow-up.

Role of the MHA (1983), if treatment refused. One could use the common law in an emergency situation. The MHA (1983) is not available to treat patients purely for alcohol problems but its use is appropriate for the delirium tremens, which is in fact an organic confusional state and so a mental illness within the meaning of the Act.

Overdose at age 81 | 06 |

The consultant geriatrician asks you to assess an 81-year-old lady on a geriatric medical ward. She was admitted following an overdose of paracetamol and appeared unwell, but did not require treatment with acetylcysteine.

1. How would you respond to the request?

2. What are the main diagnostic possibilities?

3. You discover that the patient has been admitted once previously, following an overdose, about three months after the death of her husband. She has recently been started on prednisolone for poly-myalgia rheumatica. How do you assess the continuing suicide risk?

4. Her serum urea and creatinine are elevated. She has not eaten since admission and needs encouragement to drink. She has a severe depressive illness with somatic syndrome, but not psychotic. How would you proceed?

5. How will she respond to ECT? What precautions will you take?

6. What are your thoughts about antidepressant drug treatment in this patient?

Response to assessment request. The overdose is most likely to be due to a severe depressive illness. Hence, I will make a psychiatric assessment reasonably quickly. I will introduce myself to the ward staff, and obtain a history from the medical and nursing staff and the patient's relatives, if they are available. I will consult the medical notes to understand the nature of the present medical problems, the past medical history and treatment given. I will assess the patient in private, take a detailed history of present illness, past psychiatric history and do a mental state examination. I will write down and discuss with the ward staff my formulation, what other background information is required and the treatment plan.

Diagnostic possibilities. My preferred diagnosis is a depressive illness. I will also consider adjustment disorder; cognitive impairment, either delirium or dementia; and alcohol-related problems as differential or additional diagnoses.

Continuing suicide risk. I would be more convinced of a diagnosis of depression. I will assess the current suicide risk by asking such questions as "Do you regret that your overdose did not succeed in killing you?", "Do you still think about killing yourself?" or "Is it possible that you might plan to attempt suicide again?". I will ask the staff whether the patient has attempted to harm herself while in hospital. I will establish how much contact she has with any remaining family members and how disabled she is by the polymyalgia rheumatica. Also, I will ask if anything will have changed in the social situation so that there will be more support on her return home.

Management following diagnosis. It appears that the severe depression is compromising the patient's physical health. Her depression needs to be treated quickly. The best option is ECT; I will establish if she has the ability to give consent for ECT. I will contact her closest relatives to explain the treatment plan and gain their agreement. In liaison with the geriatricians I will look at the contributory factors such as thyroid function, her medication, eg, antihypertensives, and ensure that she is on the lowest effective dose of prednisolone.

Precautions with ECT. She will hopefully respond at least as well to ECT as do younger patients. Obviously her medical problems(s) need assessment and treatment. Her seizure threshold is likely to be higher. I will monitor cognitive side effects closely and be aware of the risk of confusion.

Antidepressant drug treatment? The axiom 'start low, go slow', is helpful in this case. I will monitor her closely for side effects of antidepressant medication. She is likely to respond to antidepressant drugs as well as her younger counterparts do, but I will be prepared to wait for a longer time before she responds to drug treatment. Keeping her well in the future is of crucial importance and the best way to do this is with indefinite prophylactic treatment for depression.

Confused and not coping

A GP contacts you expressing concern about a 75-year-old widow who, he feels, is becoming 'confused' and not really coping.

1. *How would you assess the situation?*

2. *What are your differential diagnoses?*

3. *How will you assess cognitive impairment?*

4. *What further assessment would you consider?*

Assessment. The aims of my assessment will be to arrive at a diagnosis; to determine level of functioning, including safety at home; and to determine what further investigations, treatment and provision of support are necessary. My assessment will comprise a full psychiatric history; mental state examination; cognitive function assessment; and assessment of physical condition, including nutritional status and mobility. I would prefer to make my assessment in the patient's home where I can assess her living conditions and look for evidence of neglect. I would also examine the contents of the fridge. I will make efforts to obtain further information from family members, GP surgery, social services and neighbours.

Differential diagnoses. Although the information given suggests that this patient is suffering from a dementing illness, I will consider the following differential diagnoses, all of which also coexist with dementia:

- A depressive episode, if severe, might mimic dementia.
- A psychotic episode should be apparent from a mental state examination.
- Alcohol abuse: I will enquire about alcohol use and look for evidence such as empty drinks bottles.
- Delirium can be caused by acute physical illness and recent changes in prescribed medication.

The main causes of dementia are: Alzheimer's disease (insidious onset, gradual progression), vascular disease (cerebrovascular disease, fluctuating impairment) and Lewy body disease (Parkinsonism, visual hallucinations, fluctuating mental state). I will look for reversible causes of dementia.

Assessing cognitive impairment. The Mini Mental State Examination (MMSE) is a suitable tool for a preliminary cognitive assessment, although it is not comprehensive. It does not measure frontal deficit and is dependent on preservation of verbal skills. Scores of below 24/30 suggest a dementing illness but this diagnosis must be part of an overall clinical assessment. A patient with severe depression or delirium might also score poorly, while an intelligent, literate patient with Alzheimer's disease may score 28/30.

Further assessments. These should include routine dementia blood screen including FBC, ESR, U&E, glucose, LFT, gamma-GT, calcium, TFT, VDRL. CXR and MSU as appropriate. A CT/MRI brain scan should be made, especially if cerebral infarct, white matter disease, cerebral tumour or hydrocephalus are suspected. Occupational Therapy assessment can determine activities of daily living skills, and safety; community care assessment will determine the need for home care provision, financial support and related matters.

Psychometric evaluation should be made; admission should be considered, particularly if patient is at risk, possibly under the MHA (1983) if she lacks insight. Admit to a medical ward if there is concern over physical health.

Joanne is a 27-year-old unemployed woman who was referred to the psychological treatment service for assessment from the ward. She had been admitted in crisis having attempted suicide by trying to hang herself. On admission she said she heard two voices, of God and of the Devil, inside her head, giving her orders. This symptom settled rapidly without medication but she started to lacerate her forearms.

Staff on the ward took widely opposing views about her. Some felt she was very unwell and needed extra care and support while others thought she was manipulative and should be discharged. At assessment, Joanne revealed an extensive history of sexual and physical abuse in childhood. Her mother, it transpired, had watched while her partners had sex with the patient. After the men had gone, her mother would often punish Joanne by tying her up, and locking her in the cupboard for hours.

There is a long-standing history of increasing behavioural disturbance. She has never held down a job, nor had a steady boyfriend but rather drifted from one form of casual employment to another and has frequently been highly and dangerously promiscuous, earning money as a prostitute on occasion.

The assessor initially felt cold towards Joanne, particularly when she behaved seductively in the interview, crossing and uncrossing her legs and licking her fingers. The assessor's uninvolved coldness deepened into a feeling of wishing to harm the patient that included uncomfortable fantasies about harming her.

1. What is the most likely diagnosis?
2. What are the differential diagnoses?
3. What significance should be ascribed to the hallucinatory phenomena?
4. What phenomenon is being exhibited by the staff on the ward? What are its features?
5. What phenomenon is being experienced by the assessor? How should he/she respond?
6. What possible treatment approaches might help this patient?

Diagnosis. This patient shows many of the features associated with borderline personality disorder, including a long history of impulsive behaviour, repeated attempts at self-harm, identity disturbance and a history of severe abuse.

Differential diagnoses. The first differential diagnosis is a depressive illness. This may, on occasion, present with a personality disorder-like syndrome that resolves once the depression is treated. The second is a psychotic illness. Some psychotic episodes can begin with non-specific arousal and disturbed behaviour. When the patient was admitted, there was evidence of hallucinations.

Significance of the hallucinations. While these could signal a psychotic illness, they are more likely to be a brief psychotic episode in the setting of an abnormal personality. This is well described in borderline personality disorder. That they resolved rapidly on admission, without medication favours this.

The phenomenon exhibited by the staff is 'splitting'. In splitting, a patient represents people in the outer world as either all good or all bad. This allows the patient to avoid potentially damaging and confusing ambivalent feelings towards people. On the ward the patient, as a result of splitting, behaves differently towards different members of staff who, unsurprisingly, form different views of the patient.

The phenomenon being experienced by the assessor is 'countertransference'. The patient is unconsciously recreating in the assessor the same feelings as the patient supposed might have been in the mind of her mother during the early abuse experiences.

It is important not to act on countertransference feelings as though they were true. The therapist especially should not give in to the temptation to be harsh with the patient either overtly or in subtle ways. By the same token, the therapist should not react against the feelings and act in an unduly kindly fashion towards the patient. Instead, it is important to reflect on countertransference feelings and to understand where they come from. Once this is achieved it can sometimes be possible to feed them back to the patient in a modified form and this may help the patient become more insightful.

Treatment approaches. Borderline personality disorder is difficult to treat and patients require a range of different approaches to their care. The course of the illness is relapsing and remitting and is marked by recurrent crises. The mainstay of management is a unified and calm approach by the clinical team who must remain firm but caring towards the patient, avoiding both too much and too little contact. Medication and admission may both be appropriate on occasion, particularly where an Axis 1 (DSM-IV) condition supervenes on the underlying disorder. Psychotherapeutic approaches with promise in the treatment of borderline personality disorder include cognitive analytic therapy; schema-focused cognitive behavioural therapy; dialectical behaviour therapy; long-term individual psychotherapy; and, in some cases, admission to a therapeutic community.

School non-attendance 09

A GP has referred a 9-year-old boy to the local child and adolescent mental health service, at the request of his mother and the local Educational Welfare Officer. He has had difficulties attending school regularly for the past three months, following transfer to upper school. For the last two weeks, he has been unable to go to school at all. On the last occasion he was at school, he complained of a headache and became upset, running out and returning home after a PE teacher had insisted that he join in with the games lesson. Prior to this he had attended school, albeit reluctantly and with some distress on leaving the house, for two weeks when his father was on annual leave and able to take him into school. There were no significant problems in his attending school prior to this period. The chief complaint is that he gets frightened and anxious about getting a headache whilst at school.

He lives at home with his younger sister, aged 4 years, and his mother, who is receiving antidepressants prescribed by her GP. His parents separated amicably 18 months ago.

He has no other problems in going out or interference in any other activities, and he enjoys visiting his father on contact visits along with his sister every two weeks.

His mother feels that his headaches are similar to her own and are due to stress and anxiety, and she is enquiring about the possibility of his being educated at home.

1. *What are the differential diagnoses?*
2. *What are the likely impacts on the boy if this situation remains unchanged?*
3. *What are your initial recommendations?*
4. *What is the role of the mental health services?*

Differential diagnoses. My main differential diagnoses in school non-attendance are truancy and school refusal. Although he has run out of school on one occasion, this is not part of an oppositional or conduct disorder. His distress, especially around the time of leaving for school, would suggest a diagnosis of school refusal. There are no features of another emotional disorder, for example separation anxiety disorder, in this case. Comorbid anxiety is unlikely, because he settles after the initial anxiety on leaving for school. A psychotic illness is unlikely at this age, without other symptoms. There is no evidence suggesting a developmental disorder.

Impact of unchanged situation. Firstly, his current symptoms may worsen and their resolution may become more difficult with increasing time away from school. At present he is still able to attend with the support of both parents.

In the medium term, his social relationships may be affected due to his absence from school social life and peer relationships with deterioration in confidence, self-esteem and mood. This may make his return to school even more difficult, as good friendships can encourage children in this situation to return school. Transfer to a new school, as in this case, is a risky time, both following a long holiday and potential loss of friends with school transfer, which commonly has significant impact on peer relationships.

In the longer term, his education may be affected. For latency-aged children, learning is increasingly shared and occurs in groups. Homework or home tuition will not effectively compensate for this; moreover, they are likely to constitute substantially fewer hours of education. Home tuition can sometimes help if it is part of a package, eg, with a special needs teacher, including a gradual return to school.

Initial recommendations. The initial plan would be to organise an early meeting with school, educational authorities such as an Educational Welfare Officer and the parents to expedite the best return-to-school package, to which all parties can adhere, to consider any secondary gain that may have already arisen from the non-attendance, and to focus on parents working together with the school on getting him to school and handing over.

Parents should be reassured that once in school, anxieties are likely to subside quickly, despite the recent altercation with the PE teacher. Any unrecognised educational problems, which may be compounding his symptoms, should be ruled out. An educational psychologist's assessment should be considered urgently.

Role of mental health services. Intervention from mental health services is not necessarily desirable before the above recommendations have been followed. Mental health services may, however, have a role in assessing the impact of depressed mood or anxiety, to either recommend treatment or support the other professionals in urging a rapid return to school. Also, an assessment of marital or family communication problems, particularly in supporting cooperative parental management, despite their separation, may be helpful. In this case, however, the parents have a reasonable relationship.

A 25-year-old man, known to have mild learning disabilities, is alleged to have assaulted a young girl and has been charged with sexual assault. He is saying little about the alleged event. His carers at the group home where he lives are surprised by the possibility of this behaviour. They have, however, noticed that over several weeks his behaviour has changed and he has become more irritable and withdrawn. His physical health has been good. He is receiving carbamazepine for treatment of epilepsy.

1. *What are the legal issues his carers and health professionals should consider during the criminal justice procedures?*

2. *Given the above history, what specifically should the psychiatrist assess?*

3. *If he is found guilty of the above offence, what factors would you put before the court that might be helpful to them?*

Legal issues. Given that the man has a mild learning disability, the police must follow the Police and Criminal Evidence Act. He must have an appropriate adult present and ideally a solicitor when interviewed. The court may ask for an assessment and may be reluctant for him to be living in the community on bail. If an inpatient assessment is indicated, Section 35 of the MHA (1983) or remand with specific conditions may be considered. Fitness to plead (Criminal Procedure, Insanity Act) may need to be addressed. If the man is found guilty, the court may wish for advice on sentencing, eg, the MHA (1983), probation, etc, and information about him that might be used in mitigation.

Assessment concerns. Given the history of change in behaviour and the allegation of offending, the psychiatrist needs to undertake an assessment that might result in an explanation. This will include a detailed history and mental state examination with special reference to any other problems/ offending behaviours and whether the man might have developed a psychiatric illness; If he has, this might account for his change in behaviour and the alleged offending.

Other explanations of the offending behaviour should be considered including social, psychological and biological determined factors. This might include sexual knowledge, social opportunities, his understanding of social behaviour, how well his epilepsy is controlled, and so on.

Submissions to court, if guilty. A general description of the man's past and present circumstances, a brief description of his early history including special education, and a description of his general level of functioning. Also the psychiatrist's understanding of the offending – eg, if it was in the context of recent life events or the onset of a psychiatric illness. This understanding of his offending should be used to advise of the factors that might influence risk and how they might be managed and on the suitability of certain actions, eg, whether the use of the MHA (1983) is appropriate or not, the potential for community work, etc.

After trauma 11

A 32-year-old man is referred to you for assessment. He was involved in a road traffic accident four months ago in which he fractured his femur. Although he is mobilizing well he has become virtually housebound. Although the patient cannot remember the accident itself, he has told his GP that he can't stop thinking about it. A claim for compensation has been initiated.

1. What further information would you need to ascertain about the accident and his injuries?

2. At interview he says he has no memory from the day before the accident until the fourth day of hospitalization. Why might this be?

3. He tells you he wakes at 03.00 hours most nights in a panic, clearly visualizing mangled metal and flesh. He also describes panic attacks when trying to leave his house. He describes poor appetite, absent libido and sleep disturbed by pain and nightmares. He has frequent headaches, memory disturbance and is sometimes unable to name common objects. What are your differential diagnoses?

4. How would you manage and treat him?

5. What is the relevance of him pursuing a claim for compensation?

6. Three months later your patient is generally improving. You are contacted by his solicitor and asked to provide a report. The request mentions that your patient may have been drinking at the time of the accident. How do you respond?

Further information. I will consider the following:

- Were there any fatalities, or could there very easily have been any?
- Did the patient lose consciousness?
- How much pain and disability has he suffered from his injuries?
- For how long did his physical injuries render him housebound?
- Was he at fault?

Loss of memory. Until proven otherwise, this should be taken as evidence of a significant head injury. Some people suffering post-traumatic stress disorder (PTSD), however, repress memories of the traumatic event. Additionally, he might have had heavy sedation for management of physical injuries, eg, with assisted breathing.

Differential diagnoses. He has clear symptoms of PTSD and has probably gone on to develop depression. I will consider an additional diagnosis of panic disorder, probably with agoraphobia. Given the possible head injury and some nominal dysphasia, he may have suffered a brain injury.

Management. Antidepressants would help his depression, panic disorder/agoraphobia and his PTSD. Some SSRIs may be superior to TCAs in the treatment of panic attacks and are less epileptogenic. The use of either general counselling or psychotherapy is contraindicated in cases of PTSD as research suggests that both enhance the development of depressive illness. Focused post-traumatic stress debriefing, however, can relieve symptoms of PTSD more rapidly, but many practitioners prefer to avoid this in a patient who is depressed, until the depression is resolving. Specific skill deficiencies should be monitored.

Relevance of claim. Probably none. Insurance companies will routinely commence legitimate compensation claims on behalf of their clients; in his case there is evidence of serious physical injury that would normally be expected to prevent him working. With the exception of a very small number of claimants who are deliberately fraudulent and a small number whose illness behaviour changes with chronic pain, the presence or absence of a compensation claim and its success or otherwise has little or no bearing on health outcomes.

Response to solicitor. Agree to send a factual report about your contact with the patient, the working diagnosis, management plan and progress so far. There can be conflict between the roles of responsible medical officer and impartial medico-legal expert. Hence, I will decline preparation of an Expert Witness Report. This is particularly important where the claim may be in dispute for reasons normally subject to medical confidentiality.

Bipolar depression 12

A 35-year-old man, who is taking lithium for bipolar disorder, presents with a two-week history of depression.

1. *How would you manage his case?*

2. *At what point do you consider antipsychotic or antidepressant medication?*

3. *What if the patient becomes manic two weeks after prescription of antidepressants?*

Note. When discussing the management of patients with bipolar disorder, the scenario you are trying to avoid is one where the patient's medication is switched between antimanics and antidepressants without focus on the long-term use of mood stabilizers.

Management. My assessment would incorporate a thorough history, mental state examination and physical examination to determine the severity of the current episode, the risk of suicide, the disabilities, the likely prognosis and the treatment setting. I would consider possible comorbidity, eg, alcohol misuse, drug misuse or thyroid disorder. The need for hospital treatment may be indicated by a severe episode; psychotic features; high risk of self-harm judged by current thoughts and acts and by past behaviour when depressed; poor social support; and previous history of admission. Pharmacological management will depend heavily on the history of previous episodes. My priority will be to optimize mood stabilizers. Has he been taking lithium regularly? Is the dose adequate? These can best be judged by reviewing the serum lithium levels over several months. Is lithium an effective treatment? If treatment has been well complied with and at an effective serum lithium level (at least 0.8 mmol/l) over at least a year, but in spite of this the patient has experienced recurrences, then alternative mood-stabilizer treatment needs to be considered, eg carbamazepine, gabapentin or lamotrigine. If the history shows that lithium has ameliorated the severity of the bipolar illness, then addition may be sensible.

At what point other medication? The presence of delusions or hallucinations should lead to an early consideration of antipsychotic treatment in addition to the mood stabilizer. Decisions about antidepressants are difficult because of the risk of precipitating mania and possibly rapid cycling of mania and depression. The urgency of the situation, particularly if there is very poor self-care (including neglecting nourishment) or high risk of suicide, and a consideration of the effect of past antidepressant treatment may, however, lead to antidepressant prescription. Antidepressants that have been previously used and which have been effective and not triggered mania will be my first choice. TCAs may be more likely to precipitate mania compared with SSRIs and MAOIs. ECT may be indicated in severe, psychotic, persistent or treatment-resistant depression.

Manic after antidepressants. I would have hoped to avoid this situation, but will have warned the patient of its possibility, nonetheless. The risks of mania are different. Reassessment is needed as the setting for treatment may need to be changed. Mania is more likely to require inpatient care (and detention) than depression, because patient cooperation is often poor. Optimizing mood stabilizer(s) is again the main medication issue once one has stopped the antidepressant medication, but additional antimanic treatment may be indicated.

Further reading.

Bauer MS, Callahan AM, Jampala C *et al.* **Clinical practice guidelines for bipolar disorder.** *J Clin Psychiatry* 1999, **60**:9–21.

Remand prisoner 13

A 29-year-old single unemployed male, on remand at the local prison, is referred to you with symptoms of low mood, anxiety, irritability and a feeling that other inmates are talking about him. He has a history of self-harm. He is reluctant to divulge any further information.

1. *How will you assess him?*

2. *What legal information would you be interested in?*

3. *Tell me about the treatment needs of mentally ill prisoners.*

4. *Tell me about the use of the Mental Health Act 1983 for this person.*

5. *Which hospital would you consider?*

Assessment. I will take a full psychiatric history, do a mental state examination and a physical examination. I will review his Inmate Medical Record, especially the assessments by the court liaison community psychiatric nurse, prison-based community psychiatric nurse, prison staff (form 2052SH, self-harm observation record) and recent urine drug-screening reports. I will liaise with his GP, the prison medical officer and the prison staff. This will help me determine the nature and severity of the disorder, prognosis, insight, previous treatment and compliance.

Legal information. At what stage in the criminal proceedings is the inmate – pretrial, preconviction, postconviction, presentence? What is the nature of the alleged offence? Do I have access to witness statements, police interviews? Is there a list of previous convictions available? I would like to discuss the case with his probation officer. I will ensure that courts are made aware of developments such as fitness to plead or stand trial and transfer to hospital.

Treatment needs of mentally ill prisoners. There is a spectrum of needs. At one extreme we find a mild-to-moderate mental disorder, good insight, good compliance with treatment, good response to medication and support, no evidence of risk behaviour to self or others, likely to continue to benefit from treatment with monitoring by prison medical staff and visiting psychiatrists. At the other extreme, is moderate-to-severe mental disorder warranting hospital treatment, poor insight, poor compliance, little or no response to treatment already administered, risk of harm to self or to others, and a risk of deterioration in mental state.

Use of the MHA (1983). I will consider remand to hospital for reports under Section 35 of the MHA (1983) (one medical practitioner plus Magistrates' or Crown Court). As Section 35 is not included in consent to treatment provisions in Part IV of the MHA (1983), I will therefore consider Section 36 (two medical practitioners, Crown Court); there may be delays while waiting for court dates, however, and both sections are valid for three months of remand. I would prefer to use Section 48 of the MHA (1983) for urgent transfer of a remanded prisoner to hospital. Two medical practitioners send appropriate information and recommendations to the Home Office, identify available beds and the Home Office issues a warrant.

Which hospital? I will consider the most appropriate setting – special hospital, regional secure unit or locked ward – according to the principles outlined in the Reed Report [1]. I will take into account the nature and severity of the alleged offence and any previous offending, and the current behaviour in terms of aggression and risk of absconding. I will also consider resources available at the chosen unit and consider assessment by the ward team.

Reference.

1. J Reed (chair). *Review of Health and Social Services for Mentally Disordered Offenders and Others Requiring Similar Services. Volume 1.* London: Department of Health; 1992.

You are asked to see a 27-year-old woman with Down's syndrome, who lives with her elderly parents. Over the past few months she has become increasingly difficult to manage. She will not rise or go to bed until it suits her, she is moody and has also been physically violent.

1. *How will you assess and manage this patient?*

2. *There have been several episodes of disturbed behaviour when she has been incontinent of urine. How will you manage this problem?*

3. *In the end, the parents state that they cannot cope any more with her at home. What will you do in response to this?*

Assessment and management. The issue here is one of increasing behavioural problems in a woman with Down's syndrome. First of all, I will make a full psychiatric assessment. I will gather a full medical, psychiatric and behavioural history, including that of treatments, from her medical records and her GP. Then I will arrange to see the young woman both alone and with her parents. I will also obtain a full history and make an examination, looking for physical and mental illnesses. I will note her behaviour with the parents.

I will consider and clarify:

- If her behaviour varies in different environments.
- The changes in behaviour and changes in surroundings and medication.
- Patient's and parents' concerns, especially support and future placement.
- The possibility of abuse.
- The level of input from primary health care and social services.

If illness is present, I will commence treatment:

- If it is a behavioural problem, it will require a behavioural regimen.
- Possible increase in day-centre care, holiday respite and financial support.
- Change in medication may be considered.

Incontinence and behavioural disturbance. This may suggest a seizure. Has she a history of seizures or is this a new presentation? Alternatively, it may be due to mental illness, a physical illness, eg, a UTI, or it may be a behavioural problem.

I will arrange appropriate investigations to rule out a seizure disorder, check her compliance with medication and order laboratory investigations of mid-stream urine, blood sugar, full blood count and anticonvulsant levels. I will consider starting her on anticonvulsant drugs, or if she is already on anticonvulsants, altering them. Even if she has epilepsy, pseudo-seizures are still possible.

Parents unable to manage patient. I will discuss the various long-term options with the parents; these are:

- Remain at home with increased support and/or respite.
- Hospital admission.
- Admission to a nursing home, hostel or group home.
- Independent living with or without support.

Involvement of a social worker for the learning-disabled is an invaluable support. As a result of recent legislation, a multidisciplinary assessment may be required so as to allow the care manager to use his/her funds most appropriately.

Gender reassignment 15

A 34-year-old insurance salesman presents, requesting gender-reassignment surgery. He has dressed in women's clothing since childhood although he stopped this for a short period during the early years of his now-ended marriage. He is now in a homosexual relationship. He has decided to seek surgery, recognising that he has always felt that he was a woman.

1. What are the important factors to establish in the history?

2. What are the generally accepted features of assessment?

3. Can you briefly outline the psychiatric management prior to surgery?

Important factors in the history. A sense of overwhelming gender dysphoria; early dressing in the clothes associated with the opposite gender; a brief stage of fetishistic dressing, ie, eroticized dressing, in adolescence. Other features may include an intense distaste or hatred towards sexual organs the patient currently has; an intense desire to participate in the stereotypically, culturally-normal activities of a woman; and masturbatory fantasies concerning vaginal penetration.

Features of assessment. It is important to establish that a physical cause for the presentation, eg, intersex, is not present. Fetishistic cross-dressing (transvestism) may occasionally present as transsexualism. In Western Europe and North America homosexual orientation rarely confounds an accurate diagnosis of transsexualism.

Psychiatric management prior to surgery. Living as a woman for a minimum of two years is the general life test required for male-to-female transsexuals. Female sex hormones and antitestosterone agents may be administered during this period and various cosmetic procedures such as depilation and the creation of some secondary sexual characteristics may also precede definitive and irreversible surgery.

Psychiatric management consists of the identification and treatment of concurrent psychiatric disorders such as depression and social phobia and support throughout the transition process that will obviously include such matters as divorce.

A 26-year-old man of no fixed abode was detained under Section 2 of the MHA (1983) in an A&E department. He has a two-week history of increasingly talking of mystical powers, ranting about British history, cleaning obsessively, loss of sleep and undressing in inappropriate locations. On examination, he is disorientated in time but not place or person, has persecutory delusions, thought broadcasting and partial insight. He smokes between a quarter and half an ounce of marijuana daily and he uses amphetamines occasionally. He has a past history of heavy cocaine and benzodiazepine abuse. There is no recent history of alcohol or heroin abuse.

Five years ago he was admitted to hospital, from prison, for two weeks but no diagnosis was given. He has an extensive forensic history that includes theft, possession of an offensive weapon and assault. His mother was a marijuana and heroin user and has a history of schizophrenia.

1. What are your differential diagnoses?

2. How would you manage this case?

3. Is there a relationship between psychosis and cannabis use?

Differential diagnoses. My differential diagnoses are:

- Schizophrenia: he has thought broadcasting, persecutory delusions and a family history of schizophrenia.

- Mania with psychotic symptoms: he has over-talkativeness, overactivity, grandiose ideas and disinhibition.

- Cannabis-induced psychotic disorder: in view of his heavy cannabis use and because he meets most of the ICD-10 criteria such as misidentification, delusions, ideas of reference of a persecutory nature, abnormal affect and confusion.

- I would also consider the possibility of a personality disorder, probably antisocial-type due to his chaotic background and persistent maladaptive behavioural patterns.

Management. Short term management: he has been detained under Section 2 of the MHA (1983) for his own safety. He needs an antipsychotic, such as haloperidol, to calm him and reduce his psychotic symptoms. He will need a detailed psychiatric evaluation, including forensic history, physical examination, urine drug screen and monitoring of his mental state and behaviour. I will also look for evidence of symptoms of withdrawal from other drugs, such as benzodiazepines.

Further management: if he has a schizophrenic or schizophrenia-like illness, he will benefit from depot antipsychotics and input from the community mental health team. He will need a risk assessment and management. I will liaise with my forensic colleagues. He will benefit from input from the drug treatment services including help with relapse-prevention techniques. The social services could help with community care assessments, finding suitable accommodation and possibly long-term rehabilitation. With the various agencies involved, he will need a care coordinator.

Cannabis and psychosis. The relationship between cannabis and psychosis is controversial. *Cannabis toxic psychosis* is an acute psychotic illness that lasts for a period ranging from a few hours to a few days or weeks, following heavy cannabis consumption. Symptoms may include sudden onset of confusion, illusions, hallucinations, delusions, emotional lability, depersonalization, derealisation, paranoia, grandiosity, hostility, unusual thought content and temporary amnesia. Patients respond well to neuroleptic drugs and remain stable as long as they abstain from drug use. *Cannabis-induced functional psychosis* is a paranoid schizophrenia-like illness occurring in clear consciousness. It is distinguishable from schizophrenia in that hypomanic symptoms are prominent and that thought disorder is rarer. Patients respond well to antipsychotic medication. Some argue that it represents cannabis-induced exacerbation of a pre-existing psychotic illness. Cannabis may precipitate acute depressive episodes, especially in inexperienced users. '*Amotivational syndrome*' has often been reported in regular cannabis users – sufferers are often apathetic, with lack of drive, ambition, goals and direction in their lives.

An unteachable child 17

An 11-year-old boy is referred by the GP, at the request of his parents. For three years he has been at a school for children who have mild-to-moderate learning difficulties. He has tuberous sclerosis, a genetic disorder associated with epilepsy, mental retardation and a spectrum of behavioural and psychiatric problems. At the last review meeting with school, the parents were informed that their child was 'unteachable'. Over the last year he has been reported to have sat in the class, not paying attention to anything around him, in a world of his own and not making any progress. The school authorities want to send him to a school for children with severe learning difficulties because he is taking up the place of a child who could benefit from learning. How would you manage the consultation and how would you advise the parents on the management of their child?

17 An unteachable child

Every child should have the right to education appropriate to his or her developmental needs. There are a number of important issues involved here:

1) The need to support parents in their concern and in their request for help.
2) An accurate assessment of the child's strengths and weaknesses.
3) The potential role of the psychiatrist to liaise with educational and other services to find the best solution for this child's needs.

The first step will be a careful and detailed consultation with the parents alone. I will encourage them to ventilate their frustration, anger and disappointment. I will try to get a true indication of their child's strengths and weaknesses, by a developmental history and sources such as educational psychology assessments, statements of special educational needs and other assessments. Further sessions, with the child, and/or neuropsychological assessment may be required to build up an accurate picture of the child and his needs.

A number of possible reasons for being so-called "unteachable" may exist:

- Epilepsy and antiepileptic drugs should be considered as possible explanations for "not paying attention" and "not making progress".
- Tuberous sclerosis may be associated with medical complications that can affect a child's cognition and behaviour, eg, renal failure and brain tumours.
- It is important to get an accurate impression of the child's general level of intellectual abilities and any specific developmental difficulties or strengths.
- Teachers mentioned that the child "doesn't pay attention". I will explore the possibility of associated ADHD, or ADHD-type symptoms.
- The child is reported to be "in a world of his own". I would also consider pervasive developmental disorders; such children may be inattentive and have learning disability.
- I will enquire about factors at school and at home which might be relevant in the presentation.

After gathering all the relevant information, I will consider a meeting with the school authorities or a visit to the school, with the permission of parents and school. This would help me assess the child's performance in the class setting, the profile of children in the school and the school's expertise and facilities for children with special educational needs.

Further management and recommendations should depend on the child's strengths and weaknesses, his general level of development, and whether he has a specific learning difficulty, attention deficit or pervasive developmental disorder (PDD). An individual educational programme should be worked out with parents, school and educational psychologists.

Note: Tuberous sclerosis (Bourneville's disease): prevalence 1/10,000, 70% sporadic, 30% familial (with autosomal dominant inheritance). Associated with two genes: tsc1 on 9q34; tsc2 on 116p13.3. Epilepsy occurs in 80–90% of cases; learning disability in ≃60%; PDD in ≃50%; attention-deficit symptoms in ≃50%.

34

Girl losing weight 18

A GP has referred to your clinic a 16-year-old girl who has lost a lot of weight, is not performing well at school and seems to be very withdrawn.

1. *What are the differential diagnoses?*

2. *How would you assess her to help you make a diagnosis?*

3. *Assuming she has a diagnosis of anorexia nervosa, how would you manage her?*

4. *What are the indications for admission to hospital in a case of anorexia nervosa?*

5. *What would you do if a patient with anorexia nervosa continued to refuse food while in hospital?*

6. *What is the prognosis?*

Differential diagnoses. One should consider:

- Anorexia nervosa.
- Depression.
- Adjustment reaction, eg, to bereavement or being bullied at school.
- Drug and/or alcohol abuse.
- Schizophrenia or other psychotic disorder.
- Physical disorder, eg, hypothalamic/pituitary axis disorders, Addison's disease.

Assessment. I will interview the patient, alone and with the family and do a psychiatric and physical examination, looking for features for and against the differential diagnoses. I will gather collateral history from the school, if appropriate.

Management of anorexia nervosa.

- Dietician advice.
- Psychological support.
- Set target weight, weight monitoring and gradual weight restoration.
- Cognitive behavioural approach.
- Family support/intervention/therapy.

Indications for admission. Indications are: rapid weight loss, >30% over six months; severe loss of energy; exhaustion; low potassium (<3 mmol/l) or ECG changes despite potassium supplements; a home or family crisis; or a body mass index (BMI) <13.

Actions, if food refused. One should assess the patient's mental and physical state. Although patient cooperation is always preferable in any treatment regimen, there may be situations where the patient's life is at risk and where the state of starvation is preventing the patient from being amenable to psychological treatments. In such cases, use of the MHA (1983) should be considered. If the patient is detained, treatment for the mental disorder can be given without the patient's consent. This includes tube feeding, as feeding is ancillary to mainstay of 'treatment for mental disorder', ie, psychological treatments (Re: B v Croydon, 1995).

Prognosis. Mortality is 5–20%; 20% make a full recovery; 20% remain severely ill; the remainder have some degree of chronic or fluctuating disturbance. Most continue to have abnormal eating patterns; some become bulimic.

A 32-year-old man recently admitted for a first manic episode is now fit for discharge. He is a bus-driver. He would like to know when he can go back to work again.

1. What would you advise?

2. Does it make any difference that he is a bus-driver?

3. The patient turns up to his outpatient appointment a month after discharge and gleefully informs you that he has returned to his job as a bus-driver and discontinued his medication. How would you proceed?

4. What considerations need to be taken in prescribing psychotropic medication for drivers of large vehicles?

5. What are the guidelines for drivers suffering from other types of mental illness?

Advice. I would inform the patient of the guidelines under the Road Traffic Act 1988. Holders of a driving licence must disclose relevant medical disability lasting more than three months. Specifically, for major psychoses, the Driver and Vehicle Licensing Agency (DVLA) advises against driving for six to twelve months after inpatient treatment. The patient would be able to drive again after this period provided he remains symptom-free, insightful and compliant with treatment.

Driving a bus. The DVLA rules are more stringent in the case of Group 2 vehicles (large goods and passenger carrying). Longer periods of ban are imposed and consultant report is often needed before a licence is reissued. In the case of psychoses, the DVLA must be notified and driving should cease pending the outcome of a medical enquiry. The recommended period off-road is at least three years for Group 2 drivers. The DVLA will then usually require a consultant's report. There should be no significant likelihood of recurrence. Driving, while suffering from mania is particularly dangerous and a longer period off-road may be required for these drivers; this is particularly the case if the mania is rapid cycling.

Non-compliant, returned to work. This patient poses a significant risk to public. I would once again advise the patient against driving and to inform the DVLA, although this is not a legal requirement. I will document clearly in medical notes that advice has been given. If the patient continues to ignore my advice, I would be ethically obliged to inform the DVLA. There would be a risk of litigation should the patient cause an accident and injuries to third parties. It is the DVLA (Medical Advisory Branch) who make decisions about revoking licences, however, not the doctor.

Psychotropics and driving larger vehicles. Any psychotropic medication prescribed should be of minimum effective dosage and should not interfere with alertness, concentration or in any other way impair driving performance.

Driving guidelines in mental illness.
In dementia: licence is refused or revoked if there is disorientation in time/space or impaired judgement/insight. *With learning disability*: severe (no licence is issued), milder (must demonstrate adequate ability and be free of medical/psychiatric complications). *For neuroses*: no restrictions. *Alcohol*: one to two years off-road, depending on complications; medical review required. *Illicit drugs*: hallucinogens/cannabis, six to twelve months off-road, urine screen, DVLA medical assessment; opiates/stimulants: one to three years off-road, consultant's report required. *For personality disorders*: restricted if 'seriously disturbed', eg, violent behaviour, alcohol abuse. *For epilepsy*, defined as 'liability to epileptic seizures': fit-free two years or nocturnal fit-free three years; epilepsy, in Group 2: ten years fit-free and off medication.

Further reading.
Drivers Medical Unit. *For Medical Practitioners: At a Glance Guide to the Current Medical Standards of Fitness to Drive*. Swansea: DVLA; 1999.

A GP refers a 50-year-old woman with resistant depression to you. How will you manage this patient?

Management comprises:

1) Confirm diagnosis.

2) Confirm resistance.

3) Identify and deal with confounding/maintaining factors.

4) Treat as resistant depression.

Confirm diagnosis: Review medical and psychiatric records, take a detailed psychiatric history, examine mental state and physical state, order laboratory investigations and make an inpatient assessment.

Confirm resistance: Confirm that the dosage and the duration of antidepressant drug treatments have been adequate, at least two antidepressant drugs from different classes have been tried and that the patient has complied adequately with treatment regimens.

Identify and deal with confounding/maintaining factors:
- Medical conditions: multiple sclerosis, stroke, hypothyroidism.
- Substance abuse: alcohol, illicit drugs, prescribed drugs.
- Comorbidity: grief, anxiety, psychosis, PTSD, dementia, personality disorder.
- Psychosocial factors: relationships, work.

Treat as resistant depression:

i) Change the antidepressant and administer maximum recommended/tolerable dose.

ii) Administer antidepressants in combinations.

iii) Change the treatment setting (eg, from community to hospital).

iv) Augment antidepressant treatment with lithium, thyroxine sodium, carbamazepine, valproate, lamotrigine, gabapentin, pindolol, etc.

v) ECT, with a second course after six months.

vi) *Obtain a second opinion; if no alternative diagnosis given*:

vii) Try psychosocial interventions: CBT, CAT, family therapy, relationship therapy, assertiveness training, etc.

viii)*Review diagnosis.*

ix) Treatment with combinations of multiple drugs.

x) *Obtain a third opinion; if no alternative diagnosis given:*

xi) Help the patient to accept the illness and cope with it.

xii) Psychosurgery may be considered.